Lose Weight, Lose A-Fib

How Weight Loss Could Reverse Atrial Fibrillation

by

Lisa M White

Medical Disclaimer

It is an absolute condition of sale that you accept the following terms and conditions

The content of this book is for information only and is not a substitute for qualified medical advice. No person should make any medical decisions based on information presented here-in without first consulting a qualified medical practitioner.

The content of this book should not be used for any diagnostic or treatment purposes.

If you are experiencing or think you are experiencing any medical condition you should seek immediate medical attention

Whilst reasonable efforts have been made to check the accuracy of the information contained herein the author will not be held liable for errors of omissions that may be found.

Information in this book should never be used in place of qualified medical advice.

The author does not specifically endorse or recommend any of the treatments or course of actions within this book and you agree they will not be held liable in any way for any action or decision taken in relation to the information in this book.

Table of Contents

Atrial Fibrillation and Obesity

Can a-fib be reversed by weight loss alone? The answer for many patients is a resounding yes! In one of the most exciting studies on a-fib to be published in recent years, nearly 50% of the participants who lost 36 pounds were able to put their arrythmia into remission without drugs or surgery. Not only that but many of the conditions which accompany a-fib such as diabetes, high blood pressure and heart disease were also significantly improved.

More on the study and its findings later, but if you are overweight and are plagued with the miserable condition that is a-fib then these findings should give you a lot of hope. And there is more. Even if you cannot drive your a-fib into remission by weight loss alone, your chance of a successful ablation is significantly improved if you are not overweight. Being obese increases the chances of a-fib recurring after an ablation by up to 40%!

Of course, a-fib does not exclusively occur in the overweight. A-fib can occur for many reasons, in structural heart disease for example. Sometimes it occurs for no apparent reason, so-called "lone a-fib", though this term is rapidly falling out of favor as research continues. If you are under or normal weight and have valvular a-fib then it is unlikely weight loss is the answer to your problems. However, for most of us, losing weight will increase our heart health, not to mention lowering our risk of the most feared complication of a-fib, stroke.

What is A-fib?

A-fib is a very common arrythmia, and 1 in 4 of us are likely to experience at least one episode in our lifetime. It is more common in older individuals, particularly those with heart disease, but it can also occur in younger individuals with healthy hearts. It can occur as a single isolated episode – a-fib occurs after binge drinking, but the usual course is for it to occur in episodes with normal heart rhythm in between (paroxysmal) or for it to be the usual rhythm (permanent a-fib). In between these two varieties is a third, persistent a-fib which usually requires some form of intervention (cardioversion) for the heart to go back to normal rhythm.

It was once thought that a-fib was a progressive disease meaning that it would start off in short episodes and eventually progress to being permanent. However, that has been shown to not always be the case, particularly in younger patients with no structural heart disease. Nevertheless, doctors will often say that "a-fib begets a-fib" meaning that the more the heart slips into a-fib, the easier it is for a-fib to start. Therefore, it is important to do all we can to prevent that occurring and reduce the risk of complications arising from a-fib.

So, what happens when the heart goes into a-fib? The human heart normally beats at between 60-100 beats per minute in a steady rhythm which is known as sinus rhythm. When a-fib occurs the electrical signals, which tell the heart to beat regularly become disrupted. The top part of the heart's pumping system, the atria become flooded with electrical impulses making it beat very fast indeed or effectively "quiver". The bottom part of the heart, the ventricles do most of the work of pumping the blood round the body. Luckily, they do not pick up all the signals coming from the atria otherwise your heart could be beating at 300 beats per minute. But, because only some of the signals are transmitted to the ventricles and not in a regular way, the heart starts to beat irregularly and often more quickly.

The heart rhythm which occurs in a-fib is described as irregularly irregular, meaning there is no pattern to it at all. Your heart may feel like it is beating wildly, with missed beats, runs and pauses. Or you may notice nothing at all! Many people have a-fib diagnosed by chance when their doctor checks their pulse. For others, the wild erratic heart-beat makes life truly miserable. Unless you have experienced an a-fib episode for yourself, you have little idea of how terrifying this sensation can be.

A-fib is seldom life threatening

For the vast majority of patients, the disruption to their normal heart rhythm is not immediately life threatening. Your doctor will advise you more about your risks and when to go to the emergency department, but a-fib is rarely a life threatening medical emergency.

That said, a-fib can lead to complications, the most serious of these being stroke and heart failure. When the heart is not pumping out blood properly from the atria, there is a risk that it can pool and lead to a blood clot. If this blood clot reaches the brain it can block one of the blood vessels leading to a stroke. Likewise, in a very weak heart, a-fib could lead to heart failure. Both risks can be very much reduced which is why it is very important to talk to your doctors and heed their advice.

A Word on Stroke

Stroke is probably the most frightening thing about a-fib, but much can be done to prevent it. **Many people live long lives in permanent a-fib without having a stroke when the problem is treated correctly.** Your risk factor for stroke depends on many factors including age, thrombin factor in your blood, co-existing conditions such as diabetes, high blood pressure and previous stroke or TIA.

You may have heard about something called a CHA_2DS_2-VASc score. Every person with a-fib should know theirs. The CHA_2DS_2-VASc is a calculation that doctors use to work out the risk of someone having a stroke. Depending on your score and risk factors you may be offered blood thinners. Blood thinners decrease the risk of stroke significantly, although these need to be weighed against the risk of internal bleeding.

Some newer thinking regarding stroke risk and a-fib is that is not necessarily the a-fib itself that causes stroke but the company it keeps. A young person with no risk factors may have a similar stroke risk to the general population. On the other hand, an older person with diabetes, high blood pressure and a previous stroke or heart attack may have a very high risk of stroke and must be on blood thinners.

At one time doctors thought that stroke was a mechanical complication of a-fib. In other words, the longer one stayed in a-fib, the higher the risk that a clot would form. The magical cut off point was thought to be 48 hours after which blood clots were likely to occur and a patient should receive blood thinners before cardioversion. However, in the TRENDS trial, 73 percent of strokes occurred without any a-fib occurring immediately before the stroke. This correlates with the idea that it is the company that a-fib often keeps that is the issue. Therefore, doing everything we can to minimize the risk factors we have is as important as knowing our CHA_2DS_2-VASc score and working with our doctors to reduce stroke risk.

And it turns out the LEGACY study has some really good news for anyone wanting to reduce their stroke risk.

Why Being Overweight Contributes To A-Fib

On a very basic level overloading anything will cause strain. The heart is no exception. If you pile too many items into your grocery bag the bottom will start to sag and the handles might even break. Obviously, the damage is no so catastrophically obvious in the heart, but it does start to show structural changes as the weight piles on.

Structural Changes in the Heart

These structural changes make it much easier for a-fib to occur. As the body grows bigger, the heart also enlarges so it can keep up with blood demand to the body. Whilst that might appear to be a good thing, it is not. As the heart enlarges the walls become stretched and thinner. Or in the case of the ventricles they might become thicker, stiffer and unable to pump as effectively. The changes to the normal structure of the heart can lead to stiffness, scarring and fibrosis. Not only does the heart not pump as effectively but it also makes it much easier for errant electrical signals to occur.

Inflammation

Not only do structural changes occur in the heart, but biochemical changes occur throughout the body. C-reactive protein is a marker of inflammation in the body and it is significantly higher in obese individuals. It is also significantly higher in patients with a-fib. If you have additional factors which stress the body and cause inflammation such as diabetes, you have the perfect recipe for an irritable heart.

There is a subset of patients who have what is known as "vagal" a-fib. Vagal a-fib is not associated with any heart disease, comes on during resting and after eating and often affects younger patients particularly men. The culprit is the vagal nerve, a long nerve which travels through various parts of the body including the stomach and heart. If you suffer from a-fib when you have gastric issues such as wind or indigestion or after a large meal, then irritation of the vagal nerve could be to blame.

The higher the levels of inflammation in your body, the more irritable your nerves will become. They will become twitchy, act up and in the case of the vagal nerve misfire. This misfiring of the nerve can initiate an a-fib episode. Therefore, reducing inflammation in the body could theoretically prevent a-fib.

Whatever the mechanism, research has found that the risk of developing a-fib increases by 10 to 29% for every five unit increase in BMI. A-fib is ten times more common in the USA than it is in Asian countries where body mass index tends to be lower. The link between a-fib and obesity is compelling.

How Obesity Increases the Risk Factors for Stroke.

We touched earlier on the CHA_2DS_2-VASc scoring system. The higher the Chads score, the higher the risk of stroke.

The factors that make up CHA_2DS_2-VASc scores are:

Age
Sex
History of congestive heart failure
Hypertension history
Previous stroke/TIA/embolism
Vascular disease history
Diabetes history.

Two of those factors, diabetes and hypertension are directly related to weight. Type 2 Diabetes is becoming an epidemic in the developed world due to the shift to processed sugary food and carbohydrate consumption. In the USA, 1 in 10 adults have diabetes and in certain populations, Native Americans for example 15% of the community have Type 2 Diabetes.

On top of that are millions of people are living with prediabetes, glucose intolerance and insulin resistance.

Having diabetes and a-fib increases your stroke risk by around four times, even with no other risk factors.

Reversing Diabetes

For many years doctors thought that diabetes was irreversible and once diabetic you would stay diabetic for life. Recent research, including the LEGACY study has proved that is not necessarily the case. I won't tell you yet how many people reversed their diabetes in the study, I will save that pleasant surprise for the chapter which comes later. However, if you are not yet familiar with the Newcastle Diet and the Diabetes Remission Clinic Trial carried out in the UK, the results of the study found that it was possible to reverse diabetes and for it to stay in remission.

New Thinking on Diabetes

The UK based studies found that our existing thinking on diabetes may not be correct. It was thought that once the beta cells in the pancreas lost their ability to do the job of storing and releasing insulin that diabetes had set in and the condition was irreversible. If not kept in check by diet or eventually medication the condition would progress, and the complications of diabetes would set in.

The UK research found that the problem might be fat deposits in the liver and pancreas. If these deposits were reduced, in the case of the research by a very low calorie extreme diet of 800 calories a day, glucose sensitivity and normal blood sugar levels could be restored.

In the original study, nearly 50% of participants had managed to reverse their diabetes at one year. Whilst the Newcastle Diet was extreme, severe calorie restriction must be medically supervised, others have reported success with sustained weight loss and higher calorie diets.

The key to diabetes reversing diets seems to be the reducing the individuals stores of fat in the liver and pancreas. Professor Roy Taylor of Newcastle University, an expert in the study of diabetes has said that losing just 1 gram of fat from the pancreas works. To do this, an individual must lose about 10% of their body weight.

It seems then, that any diet which reduces body weight by 10% or more, could reverse diabetes.

What About Normal Weight People?

Dr Michael Mosely, a medical doctor and highly acclaimed author used the term TOFI – thin on the outside, fat on the inside to describe people of apparently normal weight who still carried fat in their internal organs. He was himself borderline diabetic but of normal weight. He found it was possible to restore glucose to normal levels by shedding his internal fat and went on to create the popular Blood Sugar Diet.

Can Everyone Reverse Their Diabetes?

Losing weight will help many Type 2 diabetics but how well it works for you and whether it reverses your diabetes depends on many factors, including how long you have been diabetic. In the original study 86% of those who lost 15kg or more put their diabetes into remission. The greater the weight loss, the higher the chance of remission.

Research has also found that the less time you have been diabetic the more likely you are to be able to reverse it. Those with the highest success rate had been diabetic for less than 2 years but at 8 years there was still a high degree of success. The cut-off point was deemed to be around 10 years but even beyond that people have reported success.

Is the Remission Permanent?

Those who put their diabetes into remission but then regained weight or returned to poor eating habits tended to have a recurrence. Those who maintained the weight loss or restricted carbohydrates for life were the ones most likely to achieve sustained remission. The key seems to be losing weight and keeping it off.

Hypertension and Obesity

If you are overweight you are much more likely to suffer from high blood pressure. The reasons for this are not fully understood, although many theories exist. One idea is that insulin resistance and other metabolic markers increase the sympathetic activity of the nervous system, leading to an increase in blood pressure. Whatever the reason, it has been found time and time again that increased weight leads to higher blood pressure and losing weight reduces blood pressure.

The Frightening Connection Between High Blood Pressure and Stroke

If you have a-fib one of the most important things you can to do prevent stroke is to lower your blood pressure. Having high blood pressure without a-fib doubles your risk of stroke. With a-fib your risk of stroke is around five times the risk of someone with no risk factors. Weight loss lowers blood pressure and puts less strain on the heart.

What Blood Pressure Readings Mean

Your blood pressure reading consists of two numbers – the first one is the systolic reading which is the pressure when the heart is beating. The second is the diastolic which is when the heart is relaxed in between beats.

Ideal blood pressure is 120/80 or less. Readings lower than 90/60 are considered to be low.

90/60 or less – low blood pressure
90/60 – 120/80 - ideal blood pressure
120/80 – 140/90 – slightly higher than normal
140/90 – high blood pressure.

Your blood pressure changes throughout the day. The reading that is taken in the doctor's office is only a snapshot. If you are concerned about blood pressure, home monitors are available, so you can monitor your blood pressure frequently. Your doctor can also give you ambulatory monitoring which is a monitor which is worn for 24 hours or longer and will automatically measure your blood pressure at regular intervals.

If one of your numbers is higher or lower than it should be that can also count as high or low blood pressure. For example, if your top number is higher than 140 or your bottom number is 60 or less you may still have high or low blood pressure.

Lowering Your Blood Pressure Naturally

Depending on how high your blood pressure is, your doctor might want to try lifestyle measures first before starting you on medication. There is a lot you can do to lower your blood pressure naturally.

Losing weight and becoming more active is probably the most effective thing you can do to lower your blood pressure. If you have heart problems, vigorous exercise is probably not a good idea, but your doctor will be able to advise you on things you can do safely which can help your heart health.

Starting off with gentle exercise such as light walking or simply just moving more can be extremely beneficial. Experts recommend 30 minutes of moderate activity five times a week but be sure to check with your doctor first if you are very unfit or have health problems.

Salt raises blood pressure so reducing your salt intake will lower your blood pressure. Processed food is full of salt and other junk additives so try to eat more natural, unprocessed foods. Salt alternatives are available but many of these contain potassium, again check with your doctor if these are suitable for you. Eating a healthy diet with five servings of fruit and vegetables a day is recommended for general and heart health – remember not to add salt when cooking!

Alcohol also raises blood pressure so keeping within the recommended limit for alcohol intake will help to lower your blood pressure.

The LEGACY Study

Drum roll please! This is the bit you have all been waiting for, empirical evidence that a-fib CAN be cured by weight loss alone.

What was the study and why it so important

To give it it's full title "The Long-Term Effect of Goal-Directed Weight Management on an Atrial Fibrillation Cohort: A 5-Year Follow-up Study" is probably the most compelling piece of research that a-fib is connected to body weight and lifestyle factors.

It was carried out in Australia at the Centre for Heart Rhythm Disorders and led by Dr Rajeev. K. Pathak. Three hundred and fifty-five a-fib patients took part in the study, which took place over 3-4 years. All the patients in the trial were overweight or obese with a body mass index of 27 or more. The average weight of the patients enrolled in the trial was 220 lbs. They were given access to a physician led weight management clinic and were later divided into three groups depending on how much weight they had lost and whether the weight loss was sustained.

The most startling results not surprisingly occurred in those who had lost the most weight. These were the patients who lost 36lbs or more. Of those, nearly 50% saw their a-fib go into complete remission. Those who did not achieve complete remission saw a six-fold decrease in the number and severity of their a-fib episodes. Their chance of achieving long term freedom from a-fib via ablation was now much higher than if they had not lost the weight.

There were many other positive body changes and a correlating drop in CHA_2DS_2-VASc scores too. Remember, ever drop in your score decreases you chances of having complications from a-fib such as a blood clot or stroke.

Firstly, 88% of the participants became free of diabetes. Yes, 88% of those in the highest band of weight loss (an average of 36lbs) saw their diabetes go into remission completely. This finding correlate with the thinking that diabetes is not a disease of a worn-out pancreas, but instead the liver and pancreas become clogged with fat causing them to be unable to regulate the glucose in the body. With Type 2 diabetes shaving an average of 8-10 years off your life, this was good news for the participants indeed.

Diabetes combined with a-fib is a deadly combination. Getting blood sugar back into normal range will help to prevent many of the nasty complications of diabetes such as blindness, heart disease and neuropathy that could otherwise occur. For many years the medical profession believed that diabetes was always a progressive and non-reversible disease. This study proves that for many individuals it is not.

So what other good news did the study hold?

Blood Pressure Reduced by Over 15 points

The participants in the highest weight loss group reduced their blood pressure by an average of 18 points. That's about twice as effective as many blood pressure drugs but without the nasty side effects.

Weight loss lowers blood pressure by about 1 point forever 2.2lbs lost. But if you are on drugs to lower your blood pressure, please check with your doctor before starting a diet and fitness regime as your medication may need to be reduced as you lose weight. Symptoms of low blood pressure include dizziness, feeling lightheaded and even fainting so need to be monitored. Whilst low blood pressure is medically more beneficial than high (mostly!) it can still cause troublesome symptoms.

Cholesterol

Not surprisingly, the study also revealed a significant drop in cholesterol for those who managed to lose the most weight. Bad cholesterol, LDL was reduced by an average of 16% and triglycerides (the fat floating around in your blood) was reduced by 31%.

Almost everyone with high cholesterol these days seems to be put on a statin drug. In the UK alone, they have become the most prescribed drug. The choice to take a statin is very much a personal one which should be discussed with your doctor. However, for many people, the unwanted side effects of statins impinge on their quality of life and in some cases the drug may not be that beneficial at all.

Side effects of statins can be quite severe, including muscle pain, digestive problems, mental fogginess and in rare cases liver damage. Statins also increase blood sugar and raise your risk of diabetes by nearly half. Added to that they can react with certain foods, so you can see why the decision to take a statin drug is one which should be weighed up carefully.

Lowering your cholesterol naturally is the gold standard and the participants in this study proved that weight loss is the most effective way to do that.

Structural Changes in the Heart

A-fib could be described as a disease of "irritable atria" and in fact the goal of a successful ablation is to destroy the irritable foci in the heart that set off an a-fib attack. For many a-fib sufferers those foci are in the pulmonary veins – the veins which carry oxygenated blood to the left atrium of the heart.

Many things can cause the atria to become irritable, valve and other structural diseases of the heart, high blood pressure, inflammation within the body, imbalances in electrolytes such as sodium, potassium and magnesium but the result of an irritated atria is often an a-fib attack.

Several things happen to the atria when we gain weight, have uncontrolled high blood pressure or heart failure. Firstly, to maintain the heart's pumping ability, the atria enlarge. Enlarged atria make it much easier for an a-fib attack to happen, one study found that for every 5mm increase in atria size, the risk of developing a-fib increased by 39%. Not only that, but in older people, larger atria may increase the risk of stroke and heart failure.

Secondly, overweight people may have enlarged hearts, and thickened heart muscles. The ventricles are the main pumping chambers of the heart, so like any muscle which is overworked, the walls of the ventricles can begin to thicken to keep up the workload. Whilst that might sound like a good idea (big muscles are good, right?) in the heart the reverse is true. An enlarged and thickened heart is much more prone to arrhythmia as the thickened walls can disrupt the normal electrical signals making the ventricles more irritable.

Whilst atrial arrythmias generally aren't life threatening, sustained ventricular arrythmias are.

Now for the good news.

In those who lost 36lbs or more the atria shrank on average by 18% and the ventricle reduced in size by 8%. The thickness of the heart muscle also reduced by 14%. In short, the heart remodeled itself, shrinking to a more normal size and making it less prone to both atrial and ventricular arrythmia.

If you are overweight and have been told you have an enlarged heart, this study should provide the inspiration and reassurance that even moderate weight loss is beneficial to the structure and pumping capacity of the heart.

Reduced Inflammation

I briefly spoke about inflammation and its role in making the nervous system more irritable earlier so anything that reduces the level of inflammation in the body must be beneficial to the heart. Inflammation is measured by the levels of a substance called C-reactive protein in the blood. The higher the level of c-reactive protein, the more at risk you are of heart disease, dementia and a host of other nasty things. In fact, it even makes you age faster!

The participants in the study managed to reduce their levels of c-reactive protein from 5.1mg/L to around 1.2mg/L just shy of the ideal level which is 1 mg/L. This reduced their risk of having a heart attack significantly.

Sustained Weight Loss Is Key

Whilst the study proved that weight loss is crucial to reversing a myriad of different conditions, one thing did stand out from the trial. One of the key factors in success is keeping the weight off. Those patients who lost weight and then regained it or whose weight loss fluctuated were not as success at getting their a-fib or their diabetes into remission.

Losing at least 10 percent of your body weight and keeping it off seems to put the odds firmly in your favor. Whilst some fluctuation in weight is normal and expected, those people whose weight fluctuated by more than 5% did less well than those whose weight was relatively stable.

The key to any long-term change is changing your habits. In the Newcastle diet, the participants did very well on their VLCD but at some point, they had to change back to eating real food again. I am sure most of them were fearful of regaining the weight they had lost and possible the diabetes coming back. This provided the impetus for long lasting change.

Similarly when choosing a weight loss plan to follow, it is essential that it is sustainable. It is not the purpose of this book to give detailed weight loss advice, that is probably best left for a chat between you and your doctor, but the key is picking something that works for you and does not feel too restrictive. If you feel hungry all the time and miserable, then something is obviously not working for you. In the chapter that follows I will give a very brief outline of some of the plans which are available and the pros and cons.

Lastly, as always please check with your doctor before embarking on a weight loss program, particularly if you are taking any medication. Some plans, for example VLCD's need to be medically supervised and approved.

Choosing a Sustainable Diet Plan

I once heard weight loss described as simply burning off more fuel than you are putting in. Well, technically that might be true, but for most of us it is a lot more complex than that. More than 50 million Americans are insulin resistant, which straight away is going to put them at a metabolic disadvantage when it comes to losing weight.

What is Insulin Resistance?

Insulin resistance occurs when your cells cannot properly use insulin. Insulin regulates the amount of sugar we have in our blood and allows our cells to use that glucose for energy. When our cells become resistant to insulin, blood sugar rises, and you are on the road to diabetes. Insulin is sometimes described as the "fat storage hormone" because it inhibits the breakdown of fat cells. This is one of the reasons that diabetics often gain weight when they start on insulin. High insulin levels are association with central obesity or the "apple" shape as it is sometimes called.

If you have high levels of insulin, you are going to have a harder time losing weight than someone who's metabolism is not "broken". And the standard medical advice of eating a low fat high carb diet could be making things harder.

When insulin levels are high, instead of transporting the glucose in blood to our cells for energy, the liver converts the carbohydrate eaten to fat. Because your insulin isn't doing the job it is supposed to do your cells are being starved of glucose and instead it is all being dumped in the liver.

Therefore, you are often hungry even after you have just eaten a meal. In fact, being overweight and constantly hungry is a pretty good indicator that your blood sugar system is broken. Low fat diets are generally very high in carbs, which make the cycle worse. If you have insulin resistance, a low carb, high fat diet is your friend. By restricting carbohydrates, the body is forced to call on its own fat stores for energy. The result, not only do you lose weight, but your blood sugar and insulin levels fall too.

Dietary Triggers for A-Fib

Before discussing some of the most popular ways of losing weight, I thought it might be prudent to look at some potential dietary triggers for a-fib. Overall, the link between diet and a-fib is not that well established, but a glance at any of the a-fib forums indicates that some people have problems with certain foods triggering attacks.

Magnesium and Potassium Deficiencies

Magnesium, potassium and sodium all work in tandem to make our hearts beat steadily and regularly. Unfortunately, the modern diet, stress and the decreasing mineral content in our soil has led to many of us being deficient in magnesium. If you are diabetic or have raised blood sugar you are almost certainly deficient in this mineral. It is estimated that up to 80% of us have a magnesium deficiency.

Magnesium deficiency alone can trigger a-fib. In a small but very interesting study reported in the American Journal of Nutrition in 2007, researchers severely restricted the magnesium in the diet of a group of post-menopausal women to about one third of the RDA. Over a third of the group had significant heart rhythm changes and nearly a quarter went into a-fib or a-flutter. These symptoms reversed when magnesium was restored.

Our modern diet is very deficient in this important mineral. Routine blood tests do not effectively pick up this deficiency as only 1% of the bodies magnesium is stored in the blood. Therefore you could still be highly deficient in magnesium and your serum blood test could come back fine.

The list of symptoms of a magnesium deficiency is long:

Muscle twitching, spasms, tics
Irritability
Anxiety and panic attacks
Tiredness and lethargy
Inability to sleep
Inability to "Switch Off"
Seizures
Irregular or rapid heartbeat
Coronary spasms
Potassium deficiency
Impaired glucose tolerance
Hyperglycemia
Tremors
Difficulty swallowing
Dizziness
Numbness and tingling
PMS
High blood pressure
Carb cravings
Craving for salt
Insomnia
Loss of appetite
Nausea
GERD
Confusion
Personality changes
Asthma and breathing difficulties
Chronic fatigue syndrome
ADHD
Tooth decay
Gum disease.

Heart tissue that lacks adequate magnesium becomes irritable and unstable. Magnesium also extends the resting period of the heart, during which it is harder for a-fib to be initiated.

Magnesium Rich Foods_

The following foods are good natural sources of magnesium and should be incorporated into your diet as much possible.

Pumpkin Seeds
Spinach
Swiss Chard
Yoghurt/Kefir
Almonds
Black Beans
Avocado
Figs
Dark Chocolate
Banana
Salmon
Nuts and Seeds
Coriander
Coffee – within reason as for some it may be a trigger
Kelp
Rice Bran

Supplementation

Magnesium supplementation has proved to be very helpful to many a-fibbers, but always check with your health care provider before adding any supplement or dietary change. Unfortunately, some types of magnesium are ineffective as a supplement – standard magnesium oxide which is the cheapest and most readily available is not well absorbed by the body with an uptake of just 4%.

Magnesium glycinate, magnesium taurate and magnesium citrate are much more easily absorbed with glycinate having an uptake ratio of approximately 80%. Transdermal magnesium is another type of magnesium which is applied to the skin. It is a form of magnesium chloride and doesn't have the same laxative effects that oral forms of magnesium do. It is generally considered to be able to remedy magnesium deficiency more quickly than oral replenishment. However, depending on the methods used it can still take 6-12 months to remedy a moderate magnesium deficiency.

Potassium

Low potassium levels can trigger arrythmia, so much so that a severe deficiency could even cause cardiac arrest. Normal blood levels of potassium are **3.5-5.0** milliequivalents per liter and levels under 3.5 are considered low.

Because potassium is so important to heart function, it is common to test potassium levels in the emergency room when presenting with certain cardiac conditions, particularly arrhythmia. Potassium is generally quite abundant in the diet so major dietary deficiencies are quite rare, however certain medications such as diuretics are known for depleting potassium stores. Therefore, doctors often prescribe supplements when prescribing these drugs. Other causes of low potassium include dehydration, particularly after prolonged diarrhea or vomiting, eating disorders, alcoholism and bariatric surgery.

Symptoms of low potassium include weakness, numbness and tingling, tiredness, palpitations, stomach pain and bloating, constipation, paralysis, frequent urination, increased thirst, low blood pressure, abnormal heart rhythms, fainting and depression.

Repletion of potassium using supplements should be done under medical supervision as too much can be as harmful as too little. People taking ACE inhibitors are usually instructed to avoid potassium supplements and people with kidney disease may need to avoid both supplements and high potassium foods such as bananas, oranges, tomatoes, peaches and cantaloupe melon.

Magnesium deficiency can worsen a potassium deficiency as the two need each other to be absorbed efficiently. In fact, if an underlying magnesium deficiency is present, it is very hard to correct a potassium deficiency. Magnesium is often administered at the same time as potassium for this reason.

Sodium

The Western diet is usually abundant in sodium, so deficiencies are rare but can occasionally occur especially when there is prolonged sweating, dehydration, vomiting, diarrhea or kidney failure. However too much sodium increases blood pressure, water retention and puts additional strain on the heart. Therefore, many a-fibbers are advised to restrict sodium in their diet.

Good Nutrition

Aiming to correct any underlying mineral deficiencies and eat a healthy diet should be the first goal of anyone who has a-fib. Bear this is mind when choosing a sustainable weight loss program. Badly formulated diets could make existing nutritional deficiencies worse and thus worsen a-fib.

Foods Which Might Trigger A-Fib

Some a-fibbers find that certain foods can trigger an attack, whereas others can eat them with no problem at all. These are the foods which have "form" for potentially initiating attacks.

Aged Cheese and Red Wine

Both substances contain tyramine. Tyramine is a compound which occurs natural in certain foods particularly aged and fermented cheeses, fish and meat. It is also found in yoghurt, soy sauce, sour cream, sauerkraut, sour dough breads, yeast extract and over ripe and dried fruit. The tyramine content in wine varies, but red wine has high levels of tyramine.

A documented case of tyramine causing a-fib appeared in The British Heart Journal in 1987. The patient who was a 60-year-old man with heart disease found that consuming foods containing tyramine would cause palpitations and a-fib attacks. When tyramine containing foods were removed from his diet, he remained free of a-fib for the 12 months that he was studied. Tyramine rich foods should be avoided by patients taking MAO inhibitors as they can cause dangerously high blood pressure reactions.

Aspartame

Aspartame, or E951 is an artificial sweetener which is used in an increasing number of sweetened foods and drinks. About 5% of a-fibbers report aspartame as causing problems, and in other studies 1 In 7 arrythmia patients reported sensitivities to it. Aspartame is reported to lower levels of taurine in the body, and as taurine is a heartbeat stabilizer this interaction could explain the arrhythmic connection.

Aspartame is in many products which are labelled as low calorie, low sugar or sugar free. These include diet soda, desserts, toppings, shakes, beverage sweeteners and even some vitamins and toothpaste.

Monosodium Glutamate/MSG E621

MSG is well recognized for causing sensitivity in some people, so much so that the phenomenon has even been given a name - Chinese Restaurant Syndrome. Glutamate can cause problems by competing with cysteine, an amino acid which is essential to produce taurine, an important amino acid for maintaining a regular heartbeat.

 Symptoms of MSG sensitivity usually start within 2 hours of consuming food containing it and include irregular and erratic heartbeat, racing heart, skipped beats, headache, flushing, nausea and sweating, numbness and burning in the mouth. For some people the reaction can be so intense that they think they are having a heart attack.

MSG also known as E621 and Vetsin is used as a flavor enhancer and is commonly used in Asian cooking and processed foods, especially crisps (chips), chicken and sausage products, sauces and dressings, and ready meals. Although many food manufacturers have tried to reduce or eliminate MSG in their products a stroll through any grocery stores snack aisles shows that it is still very prevalent in convenience foods and snacks.

 One of the most compelling pieces of evidence that MSG can trigger a-fib comes from the International Journal of Cardiology (Feb 9, 2009). The patient was a 57-year-old physician who was being treated for paroxysmal a-fib and considering catheter ablation. He then cut out all MSG and aspartame (another potential a-fib trigger) from his diet and his a-fib stopped completely. To test that it was indeed these substances that were triggering his a-fib, he set himself three separate challenges – two with MSG and one with aspartame. Each time he consumed foods containing the substances he went into a-fib within hours.

Free glutamate by contrast is a naturally occurring substance in many foods and is often considered beneficial to health, but some evidence finds that even that can cause sensitivity in some people. Foods high in natural glutamate include Parmesan and aged cheeses, soy sauce, fish sauce, mushrooms, ripe tomatoes, grape juice, gluten, malt barley, beef jerky, pork, chicken and potatoes. So, if your pizza is sending you into a-fib, you could have a sensitivity to free glutamate.

Wheat and Gluten

Dramatic improvements in a-fib have been reported by some patients after the adoption of a wheat and gluten free diet. Research has shown that the risk of a-fib is slighter higher in individuals with Coeliac disease (extreme sensitivity to gluten) than in the general population. About 1-2% of the population have Coeliac disease, yet around 30% of people carry genetic markers for the disease. Around 80 % of people with coeliac disease are undiagnosed. Symptoms of coeliac disease include diarrhea, cramping, bloating, weight loss, lethargy and vomiting, plus a host of seemingly unrelated complications including skin rashes and epilepsy.

Ingesting wheat and gluten can cause inflammation in the bodies of sensitive individuals and it is this inflammation which is thought to contribute to the initiation of a-fib. Patients in a-fib consistently have higher levels of c-reactive protein, the marker for systemic inflammation than those in normal sinus rhythm. It is important to note that intolerance and allergy are not the same thing. Allergies involve an auto immune response and the body produces antibodies in response to the perceived threat to the body.

Allergies can be diagnosed with a blood test. Intolerances do not provoke an immune response, but exposure brings on symptoms, which may vary with the length and type of exposure. Diagnosing wheat intolerance requires a food challenge under controlled conditions.

Coeliac disease diagnosis begins with a blood test for antibodies. If antibodies are found, a biopsy of the gut can confirm the disease. For anyone wanting to lower or eliminate their intake of wheat and gluten the Paleo diet has provided successful for some a-fib patients including some who were able to eliminate the disorder altogether using diet alone. The Paleo diet is described as a hunter gatherer diet and places high emphasis on meat and protein, high fiber and non-starchy fruits and vegetables. Grains including wheat, dairy products, refined sugar, salt, legumes and alcohol are eliminated from the Paleo diet.

Sugar

Since our consumption of sugar has increased we have experienced an epidemic of obesity, heart disease and diabetes. Sugar depletes important minerals such as magnesium in the body which is essential for a steady heartbeat.

A high carb, sugar laden diet can impair normal blood sugar mechanisms and set us on the road to diabetes. Since the 1990's it has been accepted that diabetes is an independent risk factor for the development of a-fib and one Japanese study found that diabetes raises the risk of developing a-fib by over a quarter.

Sugar creates inflammation in the body and people who have a-fib already have higher markers of inflammation in their bodies. For a-fibbers it pays to reduce sugar consumption as much as possible. The Journal of American medicine found higher levels of sugar in the diet increased the risk of dying from cardiovascular causes considerably. Those who got around a fifth of their daily calories from sugar increased their risk of dying from heart attack or stroke by 28% compared to those who got just 8% of their daily calories from sugar.

Salt

Whilst the body needs some sodium to function correctly, many of us get far too much of it. Not only is salt suspected of raising blood pressure in sensitive individuals by causing the body to retain fluid but it also depletes magnesium and potassium in the body – minerals essential for retaining a healthy heartbeat. Potassium and sodium are both electrolytes which the body must retain in balance to function correctly. If too much of one is consumed, the other will be released by the body to maintain balance. Therefore, eating too much salt will cause the body to leech potassium. The average diet is rarely deficient in sodium as it occurs naturally in many foods, but low potassium is a problem for some a-fibbers. There are various salt substitutes on the market which use potassium chloride rather than sodium chloride which is the prime ingredient in regular table salt. If you think that salt may be contributing to your a-fib attacks it may be worth switching to one of these but discuss it with your doctor first. Potassium based salt substitutes can be dangerous in people with renal impairment who need to watch their potassium intake. Another option is pure sea salt which retains some of the mineral content which is removed from table salt.

Alcohol

Whilst light or even moderate drinking isn't a problem for some a-fibbers, some feel the effects of even the smallest tipple. If you are one of the unfortunate ones whose heart is very sensitive to the effects of alcohol then it may be a good idea to avoid it altogether.

On the other hand, excessive alcohol consumption is known to trigger a-fib even in people with no history of the condition. This is so common that doctors have even given it a name – Holiday Heart Syndrome. During holidays and other occasions when a lot of alcohol is drunk, emergency room admission for a-fib soar. In most cases, the heart rhythm returns to normal on its own and no further treatment is needed other than avoiding excess alcohol.

Why alcohol is a problem for some and not others isn't known but it could be to do with the levels of magnesium in your body. Alcohol depletes magnesium so if you are already borderline low then those couple of drinks could just tip you over the edge into a-fib.

Whilst binge drinking is clearly a risk factor for a-fib, what about moderate or light drinking? A recent study in Sweden using a population without a-fib set out to examine how much various levels of alcohol consumption increased the risk of a-fib. Three levels of alcohol consumption: 1-6 drinks per week, 7-14 drinks per week and 14 plus drinks per week were studied. The study also looked at the type of alcohol consumed, wine, spirits and beer.

The fact that the study found any degree of alcohol consumption increased risk of a-fib wasn't unexpected. However, the level of risk and the type of alcohol drank was quite surprising. A single glass of wine per day raised risk by just 2%. However, when consumption increased to two glasses of wine per day the risk jumped to 35%. Low levels of spirit consumption - 1-6 drinks per week increased risk by 5% whereas 14 drinks or more a week increased the risk by 46%. However, the oddest set of results come with beer consumption. 1-6 drinks per week did not raise risk at all, 7-14 drinks raised risk by 11% but with 14 or more drinks per week the risk dropped back down to 3%.

Everyone is different with a varying tolerance to alcohol. Some of the effects of drinking on a-fib could probably be offset by avoiding dehydration and ensuring mineral levels are optimized. Avoiding alcohol entirely is not a practical or enjoyable prospect for many of us although it is no doubt what many doctors would recommend!

Caffeine

Many people with a-fib avoid caffeine and other stimulants as a matter of course. However recent studies show that caffeine may not be as bad for a-fib sufferers as previously thought. A study in the American Journal of Clinical Nutrition found that moderate caffeine use had no effect on atrial arrhythmias and there was no clinical benefit to abstinence. One study published in the Canadian Journey of Cardiology found that caffeine may even lower incidence of a-fib This intriguing finding revealed a 6% relative risk reduction in incidence of a-fib for every 300g per day habitually drunk! Whilst caution is urged in the interpretation of the study, one speculation is that caffeine may have an anti-fibrotic effect on the atria, thus protecting against a-fib. The good news for a-fibbers is that you probably can have that morning coffee without worrying about it

Different Types of Diet

Low Carb High Fat (LCHF)

LCHF is a way of eating that can help keep your blood sugar in check by restricting carbohydrates. The Atkins diet is probably the best-known example of a low carb high fat diet, although many dieters find the initial stage of the Atkins diet where carbs are restricted to 20g a day too hard. It is not necessary to restrict carbs to such a low level for most dieters, most people can lose weight on a diet which contains 50-70g of carbs per day.

The idea behind LCHF is to force the body to use its own fat stores for fuel. When we eat carbohydrates, a substance called glycogen is stored in the liver for use as energy. As the body usually has an adequate supply of carbs to fuel it, it rarely dips into its fat stores. Therefore, dieters on a low fat high carb diet often bemoan their lack of weight loss, they are still eating enough carbohydrate to fuel their bodies.

The body usually stores enough glycogen to last 2-3 days. When glycogen stores run out, the body must turn to fat stores for energy. This is known as ketosis – not to be confused with the diabetic state of ketoacidosis which is very dangerous.

One of the benefits of a low carb diet is that it will help to balance blood sugar very quickly, in fact most people report a significant drop in their blood sugar levels shortly after starting such a diet. If you are diabetic and on medication or insulin, it is important that your doctor is aware that you are starting a LCHF diet, so your medication can be monitored. Many people will find they need less medication on LCHF as blood sugar begins to normalize.

On this plan you will eat lean protein, meat, fish, eggs, some vegetables and natural fats such as butter. You avoid most carbohydrates, so no bread, rice, pasta, potatoes and certain veggies.

It can be quite an adjustment to get used to LCHF particularly if you are used to eating the traditional Western diet which is high in carbs. However, one of the key benefits is that when the body enters a state of ketosis (usually on the third day of the diet) hunger goes away completely.

The first week of the diet is certainly the toughest as your body adjusts to the reduced carb intake. Some people feel very tired, cold and achy, and these symptoms are sometimes referred to as "keto flu". It is very important to drink lots of water and keep hydrated during ketosis as some of the symptoms can be put down to dehydration. However, avoid drinking dangerous amounts in a short time.

Once ketosis is well underway people often describe feeling great with more energy than they have had in years. Hunger goes away, mental fogginess clears, and they have a new zest for life. Weight loss tends to occur quite quickly on this diet although the first 4 or so lbs. is probably water weight which is released when the body goes into ketosis.

The disadvantage of LCHF is that if you have a carbohydrate rich meal you will instantly undo some of the good work you have done. The body will grab the carbs and turn them into glycogen, so you will have to wait 2-3 days to re-enter a state of ketosis. You will also gain back the water weight you lost which could mean a nasty shock when you stand on the scales.

As this plan is quite restrictive it is quite difficult if you must eat out a lot or can't plan ahead. A steak and green salad is one possible eating out option, but most convenience foods and fast foods contain a lot of carbs. If you are lucky enough to be invited out to dinner regularly and you have no control over the menu on offer, then you could find yourself undoing a lot of your good work with a single meal.

Advantages of LCHF
Balances blood sugar and drops insulin levels
Once in ketosis you are rarely hungry
You do not have to count calories only carbs
Renewed energy and zest for life
Can help to reverse diabetes
Quick results

Disadvantages of LCHF
Big adjustment in eating for most people used to Western Diet
First few days can be tough
Some people are more carb sensitive than others, may need to go below 50g carbs per day for best results
If you are taking medication you need to check with your doctor
If you fall off the wagon you put yourself back 3 days.

The 5:2 diet

The 5:2 diet has been described as a "part-time" diet in that you eat normally on five days of the week and restrict calories on just two. The diet works on the premise that by reducing your calorie intake by about 75% on those two days you will create a calorie deficit, even if you eat normally on days which you are not fasting.

On a fast day, a man would eat an average of 600 calories and a woman 500. You can choose to take the fast days together or separately or swap things about to suit your schedule. So long as you eat normally (not excessively!) on the other days of the week, you should have a calorie deficit of about 3000-3500, which is about one pound of fat.

The advantages of 5:2 is that it is flexible and doable for most people. Apart from on fast days you don't have to calorie count, you can eat what you like, and it can fit around your life. You can vary the diet to 4:3 if you want by adding an extra fast day or maintain your weight loss with a 6:1 plan.

Some people use low calorie weight loss products on fast days whereas others choose to eat normal food.

Advantages of the 5:2 diet
Can eat normally 5 days of the week
Easy to fit around lifestyle and flexible
Lose 1-2lbs per week on average

Disadvantages of the 5:2 diet
Can be hard choosing healthy foods on fast days
Temptation to overeat on non-restricted days
Easy to keep putting off fast days

VLCD (Very Low-Calorie Diet)

A VLCD is a very low-calorie diet, under about 800 calories a day. These diets are extreme and should only be undertaken with medical supervision or approval. The Newcastle Diet, the diet that helped to reverse diabetes in some people was a VLCD.

VLCDs are often used prior to bariatric surgery to lose weight very quickly. A weight loss of 3-5lbs a week is average in people with a BMI over 30.

When restricting calories so severely it is very important to get the right nutrition. For simplicity and safety, most participants choose to use a commercial VLCD program which usually consists of shakes, meals and bars.

A VLCD is a short-term diet and not suitable for long term use, most commercial VLCD manufacturers recommend staying on the program for a maximum of 8-12 weeks. Rapid weight loss can cause problems for some people. Losing more than 4lbs a week can lead to complications such as gallstones.

As a short-term measure, a VLCD can be effective but it is very tough to stick to. For the first few days hunger is a real problem for many people, as is tiredness, lack of energy, constipation and feeling cold.

If you have read some of the success stories in reversing diabetes with a VLCD and are tempted to try, be aware that similar results have occurred with less drastic dietary programs. Any diet which remove fat from the liver and pancreas has a chance to reverse diabetes and although the results might not be so quick as a VLCD, it is not so hard on the body.

In the interests of disclosure, at least two deaths in the UK have occurred in people following a VLCD. Neither of these deaths from cardiac arrythmia were directly attributed to the diet but it is not known whether the VLCD contributed or whether they would have occurred anyway. Therefore, it is so important to get the approval of your doctor and be monitored throughout the time you are on a VLCD.

Commercial VLCD programs are tested to ensure that they provide all the necessary vitamins and minerals so are generally considered safe for short term use. Home formulated diets may omit essential vitamins and lead to malnutrition. If you do decide to follow a VLCD it is best to choose one from a reputable manufacturer.

<u>Advantages of a VLCD</u>
Fast weight loss of between 3-5lbs per week
Properly formulated programs provide all the essential vitamins and minerals you need
Do not need to worry about food, you just eat 3 or 4 VLCD food packs per day

<u>Disadvantages of a VLCD</u>
Can be very difficult to stick to the daily allowance.
May feel hungry, tired and cold in the beginning
Rapid weight loss may lead to gallstones
Must be medically supervised for safety

Intermittent Fasting

Intermittent fasting is not a diet. It is a way of eating which spaces meals in such a way that the body can start to use some of its stored fat for energy. When we eat, our bodies enter a "fed" state and start to break down the meal we just ate and use it for energy. When the body is not in a "fed" state, it starts to use the energy it has already stored in the form of fat. If you eat constantly throughout the day, you are always adding fuel and your body never gets the opportunity to burn its stored fuel.

It usually takes about 12 hours for our bodies to enter the fasting state. If you eat your last meal at 6pm and eat breakfast at 9am your body will have entered the fasting state for the 3 hours prior to breakfast. If you eat late and night and breakfast early, your body may never reach the fasting state.

There are various ways to incorporate intermittent fasting into your day. The simplest one is probably a 16/8 pattern of eating where you fast for 16 hours of the day and eat all your meals in the remaining 8. Alternatively, you might prefer a 24 hour fast once a week.

There are many health benefits to fasting and it has been used since ancient times to improve health and seek spiritual enlightenment. However, unlike the gurus of old, there is no need to starve yourself for extended periods to reap the benefits of fasting. Fasting for more than 24 hours can be counterproductive and unnecessary. Some of the reported benefits of intermittent fasting include:

Lower insulin levels and improved blood sugar control
Detoxification of the body and cellular repair
Reduces stress and inflammation in the body
May improve blood pressure, cholesterol levels and generally improve heart health
MAY help to prevent cancer. In animal studies intermittent fasting was found to reduce cell proliferation in several different types of cells. This could help to prevent the development of certain types of cancer. Whether this also translates to humans is not known.
MAY help to delay the onset and severity of Alzheimer's Disease. A study in rats found that intermittent fasting might prevent the onset of neurological diseases such as Alzheimer's and Parkinson's. In another study daily, short fasts improved Alzheimer's symptoms in 90% of subjects
MAY help you to live longer. Rats fasted every other day lived 83% longer than those who were not.
And of course – weight loss!

Advantages of Intermittent Fasting
Easy to do and incorporate into your life
No need to count calories of eat special foods
May lower your risk of cardiovascular disease
Improves insulin levels and blood glucose metabolism
Can help cellular repair

Disadvantages of Intermittent Fasting
Not suitable for type 1 diabetics, pregnant women and those on regular medication which needs to be taken with food
It is not advised to exercise heavily on fast days as your body might

start to break down muscle instead of fat
Some of the benefits of intermittent fasting such as improvement in Alzheimer's and neurological diseases have only been proven in animals. It is not known if these effects also apply to humans

The Paleo Diet

Paleo is short for paleo lithic or the caveman diet. It is a way of eating that mimics what our hunter gatherer ancestors would have eaten. Paleo avoids all processed food focusing instead on natural and healthy foods. Sources of protein include lean meat, fish and eggs and the diet also allows fruit and vegetables, nuts and seeds, and healthy fats and oils. Paleo excludes most forms of dairy, grain, sugar, legumes, sugar, vegetable oil and margarine. Starchy vegetables such as potatoes and corn are also not allowed. For most of us who are used to the modern diet which is high in refined carbs and processed foods Paleo involves a complete shift in the way we think about food. Different versions of the Paleo diet exist, some versions allow full fat dairy products such as butter and cheese and the occasional indulgence in red wine and dark chocolate.

Criticism of the Paleo diet has focused mainly on its exclusion of dairy products and the essential nutrients we get from them, mainly calcium and vitamin D. Whilst Paleo approved foods such as nuts and leafy greens may help to compensate somewhat, our caveman ancestors did suffer from some significant nutritional deficiencies compared with today.

Experts are divided on the health benefits of a Paleo diet, although many supporters claim that Paleo has vastly improved their health. A diet which cuts out processed food and sugar no doubt has health benefits for most people, although excluding significant food groups might not be suitable or sustainable for many people.

Advantages of a Paleo Diet
Uses real and natural foods
Avoids processed foods such as sugar
Is generally high in fiber.

Disadvantages of a Paleo Diet
Excluding dairy and grains is difficult for many people
Could lead to deficiencies in calcium and vitamin D
Because it relies on animal based sources of protein such as meat
and fish it can be difficult for vegetarians to follow
Can be expensive

The GI Diet

GI stands for glycemic index, which is a measure of how much
certain carbohydrate foods raise levels of blood sugar. The GI scale
runs between 0 and 100 with pure glucose having a glycemic index
of 100. The effects of eating certain foods are calculated in relation
to this giving each food its own number. The GI diet focuses on
eating foods with a low GI index which release blood sugar more
slowly.

You can find the various GI indices for different foods on various
websites and in GI diet books. Foods are generally divided into low
GI foods which are those which have an index of 55 or below,
moderate GI foods have an index between 56 and 69 and high GI
foods have an index over 70. High GI foods raise the blood sugar
very quickly with a resulting crash not long after eating. This can
make you feel hungry and snack more.

Low GI food include most fruits and non-starchy vegetables,
oatmeal and oat bran, legumes, lentils, lima and butter beans, and
100% stoneground whole wheat bread. High GI foods include white
bread, cornflakes, instant oatmeal, popcorn and white rice. The GI
index can get complicated, as the GI value of a food can vary

depending on whether it is cooked, whether it is over-ripe or how processed it is.

GI diets can be beneficial to diabetics or those who have problems keeping their blood sugar stable. Some studies have also shown that they may help to lower cholesterol and reduce the risk of cancer and heart disease. Heart disease and cancer are both associated with high GI diets

<u>Advantages of the GI diet</u>
Helps to stabilize blood sugar
Low GI foods release energy more slowly and help to keep you full longer
May help to prevent cancer and heart disease

<u>Disadvantages of the GI diet</u>
Need to use a reference book or chart to track the GI values of foods
Can get complex, the GI of a food can change depending on how it is cooked, processed or how ripe it is.
Not all low GI foods are healthy

Slimming Clubs

When Jean Nidetch founded Weightwatchers in 1963 she couldn't possible have predicted just how successful her enterprise would be. The concept of group support for losing weight based around a sensible eating plan has flourished and now millions of people worldwide attend slimming club meetings.

Over the past few years, the format of clubs has changed somewhat. The old-fashioned view of a dragon of a group leader berating people as they stood on the scales is far removed from the modern clubs of today. The concept of the weekly weigh in hosted by a group leader is still popular but now you can also join online slimming clubs. The online model follows the same eating plan as the group sessions but without the weekly meetings. Online clubs are great for people who find it hard to attend local meetings, who are housebound or do not want to join a group for whatever reason.

People cite the main reason for joining a club is the support of the other members and the Group Leader. Being weighed each week is a good motivator not to cheat and the various awards given out give a sense of achievement.

Each slimming club has an eating plan, generally this is easy to follow using everyday foods. The problem with this one size fits all approach is that it might now work for everyone, especially as many of these diet plans are high in carbs and low in fat. In recent years, greater emphasis has been put on flexibility and the ability to eat any food but in moderation.

Slimming clubs also put emphasis on making healthier choices with food and maintaining weight loss once achieved. Once a member is down to goal weight most reward them with free membership for life so long as they stay within a certain percentage of their ideal weight.

One downside to slimming clubs is that the membership is predominantly female. Men only make up around 10% of all group meeting members, although that number is rising.

If you live in the UK, you might be able to get the funding to join a slimming club on the NHS. Some areas are running pilot schemes to give free or discounted membership to people over a certain BMI.

Advantages of Slimming Clubs
The support of a group leader and likeminded people
Motivation of weekly weigh ins.
Awards giving a sense of achievement
Online option for those who can't attend a weekly meeting
Help to maintain weight loss when achieved.

Disadvantages of Slimming Clubs
Group atmosphere can be a bit intimidating for some people
Meetings are predominantly female
Quality of groups vary.

The Mediterranean Diet

The Mediterranean Diet is considered a very heart healthy diet so not surprisingly may benefit those with a-fib. In one study carried out by University of Navarra and the University of las Palmas de Gran Canaria, the Mediterranean diet supplemented with extra virgin olive oil reduced the risk of atrial fibrillation by over 38% compared to those following a normal low-fat diet.

The Mediterranean diet is rich in fruit and vegetables, legumes, whole grains and olive oil. The occasional indulgence in red wine is also allowed. The diet emphasizes the consumption of omega 3 rich fatty fish such as salmon, sardines and mackerel and plant-based foods such as fruit, vegetables, nuts, legumes and whole grains. Red meat is eaten only occasionally and fats such as butter and margarine are replaced with healthier options such as olive and canola oil.

Nuts are also an important part of the Mediterranean diet, with almonds and pistachios being particularly good foods to snack on. However, beware that nuts can be high in calories and fat so should be limited to about a handful a day. The grains in the diet are generally wholegrain, bread is allowed but usually dipped in olive oil or eaten dry. Wine is allowed in moderation, usually no more than around 150ml a day for women and men over 65 and 300ml a day for men under 65.

The Mediterranean diet is very low in saturated fat which may account for some of its heart healthy reputation.

Advantages of the Mediterranean diet
Low in saturate fat
Considered the most healthy diet in the world
Extra virgin olive oil may help to prevent a-fib
High in plant based foods
Anti-inflammatory, high levels of inflammation are associated with a higher risk of a-fib
High in cancer fighting anti-oxidants

Disadvantages of the Mediterranean diet
Can be quite expensive
Not particularly well defined, do not need to count calories
Possible to over-indulge in high calorie foods such as nuts

The Zone Diet

The Zone diet is a low carbohydrate diet, designed to increase a sense of fullness by eating 5 times per day. It was created by a bio chemist called Barry Sears who believed that creating a sense of satiety after meals would discourage overeating.

The primary benefit of the zone diet is that it is believed to decrease inflammation and balance hormones by being in "the zone". The Zone is a physical state in which three clinical markers – TG/HDL (cholesterol), AA/EPA ratio (a marker of inflammation) and hbA1c (blood sugar) are all within normal limits.

If this all sounds quite complicated, it is! The only way to measure whether you are in the zone is to have blood tests done at your doctors.

The eating plan itself is simpler. Balancing each meal with 1/3 protein, 2/3 healthy carbs and a dash of monounsaturated fat is the basis of the plan. To "simplify" things, protein, carbs and fat are broken down into blocks. Men are allowed 14 blocks per day and women 11. 1 block consists of either 7g protein, 9g carbs or 1.5g fat.

To follow the Zone diet therefore you will need a guide to Food Blocks and a guide to the diet itself. There is a lot of helpful information on the Zone Diet website http://zonediet.com.

Advantages of the Zone Diet
Believed to reduce inflammation
Increases sense of satiety
Doesn't cause spikes in blood sugar
Aims at achieving perfect blood test results for cholesterol,
inflammation and blood sugar
Teaches good eating habits such as portion control

Disadvantages of the Zone Diet
Can be complicated and time consuming
Can be expensive
Needs guide to Good blocks and the diet itself
Cuts out many grain foods such as pasta and rice

The South Beach Diet

The South Beat diet was created by a cardiologist and is considered
a modified low carbohydrate diet. Unlike other low carb diets
though there is no need to count carbs. The South Beat diet consists
of three phases, Phase one is designed to reduce cravings for some
unhealthy foods and cuts carbohydrates almost completely. During
Phase One, you limit fruit, grains and higher carb foods in favor of
lean protein, vegetables and a small amount of healthy fats. This is
the strictest phase and lasts two weeks.

Phase 2 in the weight loss phase and lasts until you achieve goal
weight. In this phase you eat the same food as phase 1 with the
addition of some healthy grains and limited portions of fruit. Phase
3 is designed to be the maintenance phase in which you still choose
healthy foods but are allowed occasional treats. Exercise is also part
of the maintenance plan.

The South Beach diet focuses on making healthy eating choices.
Fruit juice and alcohol are not allowed, and the emphasis is on lean

protein, high fiber vegetables and low-fat dairy. Carbs allowed are the ones which are low on the GI index.

To find out more about the South Beach Diet visit http://www.southbeachdiet.com

Advantages of South Beach Diet
No calorie or carb counting on this diet
Encourages healthy eating, regular meals and snacks
Cuts saturated fat consumption
Reasonably varied

Disadvantages of South Beach Diet
Can be quite demanding and expensive
The first stage is very difficult for people used to a regular carb heavy diet
Might be hard to continue long term

Calorie Counting

Calorie counting is probably the most flexible way to lose weight and requires no special foods or equipment other than a handy calorie counting guide. Eating fewer calories than your body can burn off is supposedly a sure-fire way to weight loss, but there are some caveats. How many calories you burn off per day depends on many factors, your sex, your activity level, your metabolic rate and how well your body processes carbohydrates.

If you have a problem with your blood sugar mechanism, plain calorie counting probably won't be as effective for you as counting carbs. Earlier we discussed how damaged insulin systems can make the body store fat. If you are eating enough high carb foods to keep your glycogen levels topped up, then your body might never access your fat stores.

The calorie needs per day for the average person.

Men aged 18-30
Sedentary: 2400
Moderately Active: 2600-2800
Active: 3000
Men aged 31-50
Sedentary: 2200
Moderately Active: 2400-2600
Active: 2800-3000

Men over 51
Sedentary: 2000
Moderately Active: 2200-2400
Active: 2400-2800
Females aged 18-30
Sedentary: 2000
Moderately Active: 2000-2200
Active: 2400

Females aged 31-50
Sedentary: 1800
Moderately Active: 2000
Active: 2200

Females aged over 51
Sedentary: 1600
Moderately Active: 1800
Active: 2000-2200

The amounts given above are the average daily amounts needed to maintain weight. As we get older we generally need less calories.

The often-quoted figure is that to gain 1lb in weight we need to eat an excess 3500 calories and to lose it we need to decrease our weekly calorie intake by 3500 or 500 calories per day. For a sedentary female over 51 that would mean an intake of just 1200 calories a day, whereas an active young male would probably lose weight on 2500. Age and sex is just not fair! The problem (or benefit depending on which way you see it) with calorie counting is that it puts no restrictions on the foods that you can eat. Technically you could eat six cream cakes a day and stay within your calorie allowance. However, you would be getting no nutrition at all.

Making sensible food choices is part of being able to lose weight and keep it off. Choosing lean protein will help you to stay fuller for longer and eating a wide range of non-starchy vegetables and fruit for cancer fighting antioxidants will avoid filling up with empty calories. However if you do want that occasional slice of chocolate cake, you can so long as you enter it into your daily calories.

Advantages of Calorie Counting
Flexible and easy to follow
No need to buy or eat any special food
Easy system to incorporate into everyday life
Does not exclude any food groups

Disadvantages of Calorie Counting
Easy to eat empty calories and not good nutrition
Need an accurate guide to calories
Need to make sure every calorie you eat is properly logged
Daily calorie needs may differ from the average

Carb Counting

Unlike calorie counting, carb counting takes no account of the amount of calories eaten, only the carbohydrate content of the food. Widely used by people with blood sugar problems, carb counting can help to balance the normal blood glucose mechanism by restricting foods that cause spikes in blood sugar, mainly refined carbs and sugary foods.

Most people eat between 225 and 325 grams of carbs per day on a Western Diet. What constitutes a low carb diet varies from expert to expert, but most agree that a low carb diet should contain under 100 grams of carbs per day. However, some people who are very carb sensitive might need to lower their carb intake to under 50g per day for effective weight loss.

We covered some of the benefits of a low carb diet earlier on in this book, and there is no doubt that counting carbs is very beneficial and effective for many people. For years we were taught that fat was the enemy, however the latest research is proving that it might indeed be certain types of carbohydrate that is the bigger problem. Most people aim for an intake of around 50-75grams of carbs per day when they first start carb counting. Fish, meat, eggs and full fat dairy such as butter and cheese are very low in carbs. Some leafy vegetables and berries and nuts are also very low in carbs. Ensuring you get enough fiber is important when you start to restrict carbs otherwise you could end up with one of the side effects of a low carb diet which is constipation. If this is a problem a fiber supplement or psyllium husks might solve the problem. It is also important to ensure adequate hydration if restricting carbohydrates.

As you are not restricted to a certain calorie amount, carb counting can be quite liberating. However, you do need to choose the foods you eat carefully, and many everyday foods might be off the menu or severely restricted. Many fruits and vegetables are high in carbohydrates – one medium banana for example can come in at nearly 20 grams of carbs.

If your weight loss is good at the number of carbs you set yourself, it might be possible to increase your carb intake a little to "tolerance" point. This is different for everyone; some people's blood sugar shoots up when they eat very little carbohydrate whereas others can tolerate far more carbs without a problem.

If you count carbs, you will probably find the mainstay of your diet to be lean protein with a few healthy low carb vegetables and fruit included. Eating more protein has the benefit of helping you to stay fuller longer but if you have kidney problems you might need to limit protein, so a low carb diet will not be for you.

Advantages of Carb Counting
No calorie restrictions
Helps to stabilize blood sugar
No processed carbs
Healthy lean protein will help to fill you up longer
Simple and easy to follow with a good reference guide

Disadvantages of Carb Counting
Will need to read food labels thoroughly to check for hidden carbs – coated meat or fish can push the carb count up a lot
Can be quite restrictive with the choice of food available
Might need a radical overhaul of eating habits if you are used to a diet high in refined carbs.

Closing Thoughts
I hope you have enjoyed this book and have learned the positive effects that weight loss can have on not just a-fib but all the related conditions that go along with it. To close I thought I would cover a few of the questions that people have asked about a-fib and weight loss and a-fib in general. If you have found this book helpful please do leave a review on Amazon so that others may find it. Thank you

Lisa White
author and ex a-fib patient

Questions and Answers

Q: But I am not overweight, weight loss won't help me.

Not everyone who has a-fib is overweight, many normal and even underweight people have it too. And whilst being overweight certainly doesn't help a-fib there are a myriad of reasons why a-fib occurs. The goal of successful treatment is to work out why it is happening to you. This might be because you have valvular heart disease, high blood pressure, food allergies, blood sugar problems or hundreds of other reasons.

There is also something called hidden fat. Some people who are normal weight have a greater than average buildup of fat around their internal organs. Unfortunately, the only way to find out if you are one of them is to have internal scans.

But yes, a-fib can and does occur in normal weight people with no hidden fat. But many of us do carry some extra weight and it is those people who will benefit the most from this book.

Q: I've lost 36lbs and I still have a-fib.

Congratulations, 36lbs is a wonderful achievement. Regardless of whether you still have a-fib, you have massively reduced your potential to suffer complications from the condition. Your heart and body will thank your efforts.

If you still have more weight to lose, there is still the potential for your a-fib to be reversed. You just might not have reached that tipping point yet.

You have also given yourself a much better chance of having a successful ablation (if you so choose) by losing the weight. You have reduced the chances of complications during the procedure and improved your chances of long term return to normal heart rhythm.

Q: Do I need my doctors consent to lose weight?

You need to speak to your doctor before embarking on any weight loss program. Not only will they be able to give you help and support, but they will be able to monitor any drugs you are on to ensure you are still on the correct dosage. Some diets for example might lower blood sugar very quickly, which if you are already on medication to lower your blood glucose might give you nasty side effects or be dangerous. Always follow your doctor's advice.

Q.Will I be able to come off blood-thinners if I lose weight and my a-fib reverses?

Again, this is a question which needs to be discussed between you and your doctor. Never stop taking any prescribed drug, especially blood thinners without the consent of your doctor.

Q. Can some foods trigger a-fib?

Yes, see the chapter on dietary triggers. In some people, some foods absolutely can precipitate an attack. If you think your a-fib might be dietary related, then try to keep a diary of everything you eat to see if there is any correlation between episodes and food.

Q. All this is based on just one report though.

This was a thorough study involving over 1400 patients with a-fib.

It was followed up over a five-year period. It confirmed what doctors had suspected for a while, that a-fib responded to long term and sustained weight loss. This is something that a-fib specialists had seen many times, that people who could lose weight and keep it off, often made a-fib go away. If you search the internet you will find many other studies that have similar results, but this was the most prominent piece of research which confirmed the hypothesis.

Q. You said you were an ex a-fib patient. How did you get your cure?

Yes, I used to suffer from a-fib and as such I want to do everything I can to help other people find their cure like I did. I was diagnosed with lone paroxysmal a-fib 17 years ago when I was 31. I was a bit of a medical mystery because even though my rhythm strips clearly showed a-fib, no doctor could work out why. I was kept in hospital after that first episode for three days while the doctors did every test they possibly could. My heart was healthy, echo was perfect, I was not the typical a-fib patients, 31, female and healthy. But I had a-fib. Back then catheter ablation was in its infancy and the only other hope for a permanent cure was the MAZE procedure which no doctor would carry out on someone with a healthy heart. So, I decided to solve my own medical mystery. After a lot of research, I found that my problem was magnesium deficiency, caused primarily by my bad diet and huge amounts of stress. Replenishing my magnesium stores worked quickly for me, and I have since found out it has done for many others. One interesting study found that women who ate a restricted magnesium diet were much more prone to go into a-fib and have other heart disturbances which resolved quickly by replacing the magnesium lost. If you are interested in the connection between low magnesium levels and a-fib, may I point you to the writings of the excellent Dr Carolyn Dean who has done a lot of work in this area. Even though I no longer have a-fib I am still interested in helping others with this condition.

Even though a-fib is not generally considered life threatening I know it had a massive impact on my life, spiraling me into despair and depression. If I can help anyone through my books I would consider it an honor.

Q. Can I lose weight too quickly?

That is an interesting question. On one hand patients undergoing bariatric surgery often lose a lot of weight very quickly with seemingly no ill effects. On the other hand, dieticians tell us that 1-2lbs per week is a sensible and safe amount of weight to lose per week. Rapid weight loss sometimes results in the loss of muscle rather than fat, and as the heart is a muscle it is probably a good idea for a-fib patients to err on the side of caution and not lose too fast. The important factor that came from the LEGACY study is that weight loss must be sustained for the most effective results. Therefore, losing 5lbs one week and gaining 2 the next would not get the same results as a steady 1-2lb weight loss. However, weight does fluctuate somewhat from week to week depending on many factors like water retention, but the take home message seems to be your weight loss chart should have a steady downward gradient and not look like the ECG of an a-fib patient!

Q. Which diet would work best for me?

That is totally a personal choice. I have outlined some of the most popular dietary strategies in this book but there are many more. Which diet you choose is largely up to you so long as you get good nutrition and find the plan sustainable.

Q. My doctor says my diabetes is not reversible and I will have it for life. Is that true?

For many years doctors saw diabetes as a progressive and not reversible condition but opinion is changing. The results from the LEGACY study are proving that in some cases, diabetes can be reversed. Type 2 diabetes could be a symptom of too much fat in the liver and pancreas rather than the destruction of the beta cells of the pancreas as previously thought. Further studies are underway to prove this hypothesis.

In the meantime, diabetes forums are full of people who have claimed to reverse diabetes and even my doctor now believes that the condition is reversible. A low carb diet will drop blood sugar levels very quickly for many people, but the test is how the body responds when given a glucose load. If the blood sugar remains at normal levels, then the condition might be considered reversed. However, whether blood sugar levels will remain normal waits to be seen. If you start eating a lot of high carb foods and overload the liver and pancreas with fat, blood sugar levels will start to rise again.

Q. I have lost weight and my a-fib seems to have gone away. Will it come back?

No-one has a crystal ball but if you have successfully reversed your a-fib and you maintain your weight loss you have given yourself the best possible chance of reducing any of the complications of a-fib. There is no point worrying about what may or may not happen in the future. Focus instead on enjoying your a-fib free life.

Made in the USA
Las Vegas, NV
23 April 2024

89047489R00042